USING ASHWAGANDHA FOR BEGINNERS

A Natural Guide To Stress Relief, Energy Boost, And Hormonal Balance For Wellness Beginners

JACK MURILLO

Contents

INTRODUCTION

Ashwagandha, often referred to as the "queen of herbs," is a revered adaptogen deeply rooted in the heart of Ayurveda—India's ancient system of natural healing.

Known scientifically as Withania somnifera, this potent herb carries a legacy of over 3,000 years, celebrated for its ability to harmonize the body and mind.

For beginners seeking a natural path to balance and vitality, Ashwagandha is an ideal starting point, offering gentle yet profound support for overall well-being.

Definition and Historical Context

Ashwagandha translates to "smell of the horse" in Sanskrit, alluding to its distinct aroma and the strength it imparts.

This herb has been used for centuries in traditional medicine to enhance stamina, support cognitive health, and build resilience against stress. Historical Ayurvedic texts praise its rejuvenating qualities, considering it a Rasayana—a class of remedies aimed at promoting longevity and vitality.

Origin and Cultural Importance

Native to the arid regions of India, parts of the Middle East, and North Africa, Ashwagandha has held a sacred place in cultural practices and wellness traditions.

In Indian households, it's as much a symbol of natural health as it is a remedy for the weary. Farmers carefully tend to its hardy, resilient plants, which thrive in challenging climates—a metaphor for the herb's own ability to help humans withstand life's pressures.

In Ayurveda, it has been used to balance Vata and Kapha doshas and is often prescribed for calming the nervous system, restoring physical energy, and revitalizing the spirit. Its cultural significance extends beyond wellness; Ashwagandha is a living bridge to ancient wisdom.

Why Beginners Should Explore Ashwagandha

Key Benefits

Stress Relief and Mental Clarity: Modern life demands a lot from our minds, and Ashwagandha has been scientifically validated for its ability to lower cortisol levels—the hormone linked to stress.

Energy and Endurance: Whether you're looking to boost your fitness journey or simply have more energy to get through your day, Ashwagandha can be your natural ally.

Cognitive Support: Studies suggest it may enhance memory, focus, and learning ability, making it a favorite among professionals and students alike.

Immunity Boost: With its natural antioxidant properties, Ashwagandha strengthens the immune system, helping you resist common ailments.

Ashwagandha is beginner-friendly. Available in powders, capsules, or teas, it integrates seamlessly into daily routines.

Its gentle, adaptogenic nature means it works with your body's unique needs, making it suitable for nearly everyone.

Unlike synthetic supplements, it's a plant-based remedy that offers balance without side effects when used appropriately.

Website Idea For Ashwagandha Beginners

Name: AshwaPath: The Beginner's Guide to Ashwagandha

Mission: Empowering individuals to embark on a journey of natural wellness through Ashwagandha.

Features:
Educational Blogs: Dive deep into the science and history of Ashwagandha.

Product Reviews: Explore trusted Ashwagandha supplements.

Usage Guides: Step-by-step advice for beginners on how to incorporate Ashwagandha into daily life.

Community Forum: Connect with others exploring the benefits of this incredible herb.

Expert Q&A: Insights from Ayurvedic practitioners and modern wellness experts.

This digital resource could be a welcoming space for anyone eager to learn about this herb's incredible benefits while respecting its rich cultural roots.

CHAPTER 1

Understanding Ashwagandha

Ashwagandha, often called the "Indian Ginseng," is a cornerstone of traditional Ayurvedic medicine, revered for its adaptogenic properties.

Derived from the root and berries of the plant Withania somnifera, it has been used for centuries to enhance vitality, reduce stress, and improve overall well-being.

Brief History Of Ashwagandha

Ashwagandha's roots trace back to ancient India, where it was considered a "Rasayana" (rejuvenative herb). Sanskrit texts describe it as a remedy to increase strength and stamina, likening its effects to that of a horse.

Over millennia, Ashwagandha gained popularity for its role in promoting longevity and balancing the body's natural functions.

Quote: "Ashwagandha: a timeless remedy blending the wisdom of Ayurveda with the needs of modern life."

Natural Vs. Artificial Ashwagandha

Key Differences
Source:

Natural Ashwagandha is harvested directly from organically cultivated Withania somnifera plants.

Artificial Ashwagandha refers to synthesized versions or extracts augmented with other compounds to enhance potency or shelf life.

Nutritional Profile:
Natural forms retain their full spectrum of phytochemicals, while artificial forms may isolate specific active ingredients like withanolides.

Effectiveness:
Natural Ashwagandha works holistically, addressing multiple health needs. Artificial options can target specific issues more effectively but may lose some synergistic benefits.

Similarities and Overlaps

Both types aim to deliver adaptogenic benefits, helping the body manage stress and balance hormones. They are available in forms such as capsules, powders, and teas.

The Secret Behind Artificial And Natural Forms
Artificial forms often incorporate advanced extraction techniques, increasing withanolide content while reducing impurities. On the other hand, natural Ashwagandha embraces the wisdom of its whole-root form, delivering a balanced effect rooted in tradition.

Example Recipes:

Natural Ashwagandha Milk Tonic:
Blend 1 tsp Ashwagandha powder with warm milk, honey, and a pinch of cardamom.

Artificial Ashwagandha Smoothie:
Use 500mg encapsulated extract in a green smoothie with spinach, banana, and almond milk.

Characteristics Of The Ashwagandha Plant

Botanical Features
Ashwagandha is a small shrub with yellow-green flowers and bright red berries. Its roots have a distinct earthy aroma, hinting at its name, which translates to "smell of a horse."

Cultivation and Growth
Grows in dry, subtropical climates.

Thrives in well-drained soil with plenty of sunlight.

Harvested between 150-180 days after planting.

Diagram: Anatomy of the Ashwagandha Plant

Roots: Medicinal part used for stress and energy.

Berries: Sometimes used for culinary and medicinal purposes.

Leaves: Have mild therapeutic properties.

Types And Variations Of Ashwagandha

Different Species and Their Uses
Withania somnifera: Primary medicinal species.

Withania coagulans: Used in traditional cheese-making and as a digestive aid.

Capsules: Encapsulated powders or extracts.

Powders: Pure root or leaf powders.

Teas: Infusions combining Ashwagandha with other calming herbs.

Column Table: Quick Comparison of Natural vs. Artificial Ashwagandha

Aspect	Natural Ashwagandha	Artificial Ashwagandha
Source	Organic, whole plant	Lab-extracted, isolated compounds
Potency	Holistic effect with diverse phytochemicals	Enhanced potency for targeted issues
Cost	Generally affordable	Can be pricier due to extraction processes
Preparation	Requires brewing or mixing	Ready-to-use capsules or tablets
Suitability	Ideal for holistic wellness seekers	Better for specific, fast-acting benefits

Reproduction & Distribution Process

Propagation:
Seeds are planted in prepared beds. Clonal propagation can be used for uniform quality.

Harvesting:
Roots are washed, cut, and dried under controlled conditions to preserve phytochemicals.

Processing:
For natural forms: Powdered or dried whole.

For artificial forms: Extracted and standardized to desired potency.

Distribution:
Packaged into consumer-friendly products like capsules, powders, and teas.

Purpose Of Studying Ashwagandha To Become An Expert

Becoming proficient in Ashwagandha involves understanding its cultivation, preparation, and applications. Expertise allows professionals to:

Formulate effective health products.

Guide consumers toward appropriate choices.

Advocate for sustainable farming practices.

Visual Representation (Diagram Map)

A labeled infographic displaying the Ashwagandha plant's parts, cultivation steps, and product lifecycle, from planting seeds to consumer packaging.

CHAPTER 2

Benefits And Uses Of Ashwagandha

Brief History Of Ashwagandha

Ashwagandha, also known as "Indian ginseng" or Withania somnifera, has been revered in Ayurveda for centuries. Originating in India and Africa, its name translates to "smell of horse," symbolizing the herb's strength-giving properties.

Traditional healers used Ashwagandha to rejuvenate the body, promote longevity, and enhance mental clarity. Today, its benefits are recognized worldwide for stress management, energy enhancement, and overall wellness.

Benefits And Uses Of Ashwagandha

Ashwagandha's versatility makes it an essential adaptogen. Below is a structured outline of its key benefits, with detailed explanations and a recipe for each use.

Benefit	Description	Example Recipe
Stress Relief	Reduces cortisol levels, calming the nervous system.	**Stress Relief Tea**: Steep 1 tsp Ashwagandha powder in hot water; add honey.
Improved Sleep	Promotes relaxation and improves sleep quality.	**Golden Milk**: Mix 1 cup warm milk, 1 tsp Ashwagandha, turmeric, and cinnamon.

Enhanced Energy	Boosts stamina and combats fatigue.	**Morning Smoothie**: Blend Ashwagandha, banana, almond milk, and chia seeds.
Boosted Immunity	Enhances white blood cell activity and resilience against infections.	**Immunity Tonic**: Combine Ashwagandha, ginger, and lemon juice in warm water.
Hormonal Balance	Supports endocrine function and fertility.	**Balancing Tea**: Brew Ashwagandha and licorice root with a dash of honey.

Top Reasons To Use Ashwagandha

Stress Relief

Chronic stress wreaks havoc on physical and mental health. Ashwagandha lowers cortisol levels, reducing anxiety and tension.

Visual Aid:

Diagram: A graph showing cortisol levels before and after regular Ashwagandha use.

Improved Sleep

Insomnia or poor sleep affects overall health. Ashwagandha works as a natural sedative to promote deep, restorative sleep.

Enhanced Energy Levels

By supporting the adrenal glands, Ashwagandha combats chronic fatigue and increases endurance.

Boosted Immunity

A potent antioxidant, it strengthens the immune system, making the body more resilient to infections.

Hormonal Balance

Especially beneficial for women during menopause or irregular cycles, Ashwagandha regulates hormonal activity.

Ashwagandha for Specific Health Issues

Health Concern	Role of Ashwagandha	How to Use
Anxiety and Mental Health	Alleviates anxiety and depression by enhancing serotonin production.	**Calming Capsule**: Take 300 mg Ashwagandha daily.
Physical Endurance	Enhances athletic performance and muscle recovery.	**Post-Workout Shake**: Add 1 tsp Ashwagandha to a protein shake.
Cognitive Function	Improves focus, memory, and mental clarity.	**Brain Boost Tea**: Brew with Brahmi and green tea.

Safety And Dosage Recommendations

Understanding the correct usage of Ashwagandha is vital for its effectiveness.

Who Should Avoid Ashwagandha?

Pregnant and breastfeeding women.

Individuals with autoimmune diseases like lupus or rheumatoid arthritis.

Those on thyroid medication, as Ashwagandha may interfere with its action.

Common Side Effects

Mild nausea.

Stomach upset.

Rare allergic reactions.

Dosage Guidelines	Form	Recommended Amount
Stress/Anxiety Relief	Capsule	300–600 mg daily.
Sleep Improvement	Powder	1/2–1 tsp with milk before bed.
Energy Boost	Tincture	2–4 drops diluted in water, twice a day.

Purpose Of Studying Ashwagandha To Become An Expert

Mastering the uses of Ashwagandha opens doors to holistic wellness expertise. Professionals in herbal medicine, wellness coaching, or Ayurveda gain profound knowledge to guide others effectively. The study involves:

Understanding Ashwagandha's biochemical properties.

Learning preparation techniques for maximum potency.

Educating others about its safe integration into daily life.

Cultivation
Grown in arid regions of India.

Requires well-drained soil and ample sunlight.

Harvesting
Roots are extracted, cleaned, and dried.

Processing
Dried roots are powdered, encapsulated, or turned into tinctures.

Distribution
Packaged products are distributed through health stores and online platforms.

Visual Map

Diagram:
Illustrate the cycle from cultivation → processing → consumption with labels.

Quote To Ponder
"Ashwagandha is not just a herb; it is nature's way of gifting balance, strength, and calmness to the modern soul."

CHAPTER 3

Challenges For Beginners

Common Hurdles

Starting your journey with ashwagandha can feel overwhelming due to the vast information available. Beginners often grapple with uncertainties regarding its benefits, dosage, and quality.

Recipe to Address:
Content Plan:

Explain the importance of researching sources for authentic ashwagandha products.

Include step-by-step guidance for first-time buyers: labels to look for, certifications to check, and ensuring the product is free of harmful additives.

Discuss the adaptation period for beginners and suggest ways to monitor one's body response.

Misconceptions

Misconceptions around ashwagandha abound, such as the belief that it's a miracle cure or only suitable for stress relief.

Recipe to Address:
Content Plan:

Highlight common myths and their corrections. For instance, while it supports stress management, it's also a powerful adaptogen promoting overall well-being.

Include quotes from experts and scientific references to back up claims.

Introduce a myth vs. reality column for clarity.

Overdose and Misuse Risks

5 Reasons You Should Not Use Ashwagandha

Lack of Professional Advice: Self-diagnosing and self-prescribing can lead to misuse.

Overdose Risks: Taking more than recommended might lead to gastrointestinal distress, headaches, or drowsiness.

Mixing with Medications: Ashwagandha may interact negatively with certain medications.

Potential Allergies: Sensitivities may cause skin rashes or respiratory issues.

Unsuitable Conditions: People with autoimmune diseases, thyroid imbalances, or during pregnancy should avoid it.

Recipe to Address:
Content Plan:

Offer practical tips to prevent overdosing (e.g., using a calibrated spoon).

Provide a list of contraindications with actionable advice, such as consulting a physician.

Overcoming Challenges As A Beginner

Safe Practices

Adopting safe practices ensures a positive experience.

Recipe to Address:
Content Plan:

Detail the importance of starting with low doses and gradually increasing based on tolerance.

Suggest timing for consumption: morning for energy or evening for relaxation.

Incorporate a weekly journal template to track effects.

Consultation With Professionals

Expert guidance can save beginners from many hurdles.

Recipe to Address:
Content Plan:

Provide a guide to finding reliable healthcare providers with experience in herbal remedies.

Share questions to ask a professional to ensure safe usage.

Clear Map/Diagram for Better Understanding

Visual Example

A flowchart or timeline could outline the beginner's journey:

Week 1-2: Begin with 300mg per day, focus on observing body responses.

Week 3-4: Gradually increase to 600mg (if no adverse effects occur).

Month 2+: Decide on long-term use based on goals (stress relief, energy).

Below is a conceptual map for Ashwagandha Beginners:

Left Side: Safety First

Dosage: Start small.

Check for allergies.

Avoid during pregnancy or auto-immune conditions.

Right Side: Maximizing Benefits

Pair with mindfulness exercises.

Balance with a healthy diet.

Incorporate ashwagandha in tea, smoothies, or capsules.

Column Table Example

Aspect	Tips/Details	Example
Starting Dose	Begin with 300mg/day	Use a kitchen scale for

		accuracy
Tracking Progress	Maintain a journal for mood, energy, and sleep changes	Write daily notes in a notebook
Identifying Products	Choose certified organic and lab-tested products	Look for USDA-certified labels
Professional Advice	Consult with an herbalist or naturopath	Ask about interaction with meds
Avoiding Risks	Don't mix with alcohol or sedatives	Take at least 2 hours apart

Background Information And History

Ashwagandha, also known as Withania somnifera, is a revered herb in Ayurveda with a history spanning over 3,000 years.

Native to India, the Middle East, and parts of Africa, it has been traditionally used to enhance vitality, reduce stress, and improve cognitive function. Today, its adaptogenic properties are supported by modern research.

Website Example:

A page titled "Your Beginner's Guide to Ashwagandha" with sections:

CHAPTER 4

Crafting A Business Around Ashwagandha

Building a business around ashwagandha, a powerful adaptogenic herb, involves blending ancient wisdom with modern innovation.

From crafting therapeutic products to creating niche markets, this chapter unravels the transformative potential of ashwagandha. Let us dive deeply into its lucrative opportunities.

What Is An Ashwagandha Craft Business?

An Ashwagandha Craft Business focuses on utilizing this herb to produce artisanal, therapeutic, and lifestyle-enhancing products.

It ranges from health supplements, teas, and oils to handmade cosmetics and sustainable packaging.

Recipe for Understanding
Vision: Build a brand rooted in wellness.

Ingredients:

Knowledge of ashwagandha benefits.

Small-scale production techniques.

An understanding of global wellness trends.

Process:

Research applications and therapeutic values.

Design product prototypes (e.g., ashwagandha tinctures, calming teas, organic soaps).

Identify potential target markets.

Quote: "A business grounded in nature is a business destined to thrive."

Exploring Niche Opportunities
Ashwagandha offers a spectrum of niche opportunities:

Herbal Skincare Products: Infused soaps, serums, and face masks.

Health Supplements: Capsules, powders, and herbal teas.

Artisanal Gifts: Handcrafted ashwagandha-infused candles or wellness kits.

Food and Beverage: Nutritional bars and infused chocolates.

Lifestyle Goods: Yoga mats paired with adaptogenic teas.

Practical Example

Create a "Stress Relief Kit" containing:

Ashwagandha tea blends.

Bath bombs infused with ashwagandha oil.

A guide to mindful living.

A Complete Ashwagandha Business Plan For Beginners

This section presents an actionable plan for beginners to launch an ashwagandha business.

Market Research
Assess consumer interest.

Analyze competitors in the herbal product market.

Sourcing and Distribution
Partner with organic farms for ethically sourced ashwagandha.

Build a small distribution network.

Branding and Marketing
Develop a unique logo and eco-conscious packaging.

Promote products via social media and wellness influencers.

Key Table: Business Plan Breakdown

Step	Details	Example
Market Research	Analyze demand in urban wellness markets	Surveys targeting yoga studios
Product Prototypes	Develop samples for target markets	Ashwagandha green tea
Sourcing	Partner with local organic farms	Ethical ashwagandha cultivators

| Branding | Create a name/logo focusing on nature | "AdaptLife Naturals" |
| Marketing | Utilize Instagram influencers | Wellness micro-bloggers |

Distribution And Reproduction Processes

Reproduction Process
Use traditional methods for consistency (e.g., low-heat drying of ashwagandha roots to preserve potency).

Implement modern tools for scalability.

Distribution
Collaborate with eco-friendly delivery services.

Leverage digital platforms (Amazon, Etsy).

Sustainable Practices
The backbone of a thriving ashwagandha business is sustainability:

Ethical Sourcing: Partner with farms adhering to organic certifications.

Eco-friendly Packaging: Use biodegradable materials.

Community Support: Work with small-scale farmers.

Quote: "Sustainability is not just a practice; it's a promise to the planet."

Quality Control
Ensuring product excellence through:

Rigorous testing for potency and purity.

Certifications for organic and fair-trade standards.

Regular audits of supply chain practices.

Visual Map: A Beginner's Roadmap to Ashwagandha Business Success

Start: Passion for wellness → Education on ashwagandha.

Develop: Research niches → Create prototypes.

Grow: Launch a small-scale production unit → Build partnerships.

Expand: Scale sustainably → Embrace innovation.

Creative Craft Business With Ashwagandha

Harness creativity to offer customers unique products with a therapeutic edge. For instance, handcrafted ashwagandha soaps can serve dual purposes: skin therapy and aromatherapy.

DIY Recipe: Ashwagandha Soap
Ingredients:

Melt-and-pour soap base.

Ashwagandha powder (2 tbsp).

Essential oils (e.g., lavender).

Steps:

Melt the soap base.

Add ashwagandha and essential oils.

Pour into molds and let cool.

By emphasizing the harmony of wellness, sustainability, and innovation, this guide transforms ashwagandha into more than just an herb—it becomes the foundation of a flourishing business.

CHAPTER 5

Care And Maintenance

"To cultivate the best from nature, we must nurture it with care and respect."

Ashwagandha, also known as Withania somnifera, is a powerful herb revered for centuries in Ayurvedic medicine. For beginners, understanding the care and maintenance of Ashwagandha ensures you cultivate a robust, healthy plant and extract its maximum benefits.

Key Components Of Care And Maintenance

Pruning and Weeding:
Regularly remove weeds to prevent nutrient competition.

Prune dead or yellowing leaves to encourage healthy growth.

Pest Control:
Use organic neem oil sprays to manage pests without chemical residues.

Fertilizing:
Incorporate compost or organic fertilizers once a month during the growing season.

Sunlight:
Ensure 6-8 hours of direct sunlight daily. Place pots in sunny spots for optimal growth.

Growing Ashwagandha At Home

"A garden is not only for plants to grow but also for the soul to heal."

Growing Ashwagandha at home allows you to cultivate its medicinal roots personally. The joy of tending to this plant is coupled with the assurance of organic and fresh produce.

Step-By-Step Guide

Prepare the Soil:
Use well-drained sandy or loamy soil enriched with compost.

Planting:
Sow seeds 1 cm deep, spaced 10 inches apart, ensuring room for root expansion.

Watering:
Water sparingly; overwatering may cause root rot.

Harvesting:
Harvest roots after 5-6 months when the plant's leaves begin to dry.

Recipes for Ashwagandha-based Wellness Drinks:

Ashwagandha Tea:
Ingredients: 1 tsp Ashwagandha powder, 1 cup water, honey.

Steps: Boil water, mix in powder, simmer for 5 minutes, strain, and add honey.

Golden Milk:

Ingredients: 1 tsp Ashwagandha powder, 1 cup milk, turmeric, and a pinch of black pepper.

Steps: Warm milk, mix all ingredients, and enjoy before bed for restful sleep.

Soil, Water, and Climate Requirements

"Nature's blueprint must be respected to unlock its secrets."

Key Requirements:
Soil:

Sandy, well-drained soil with a pH of 6.0-7.5 is ideal.

Water:

Moderate irrigation, preferably once every 7-10 days in well-drained soil.

Climate:

Thrives in warm, dry climates, with temperatures between 20-35°C (68-95°F).

Maintaining Product Quality In Business

"Consistency is the cornerstone of excellence."

For businesses, maintaining the quality of Ashwagandha products ensures customer trust and long-term success.

Steps to Maintain Quality:
Controlled Drying:

Dry roots in shade to retain their active compounds. Avoid direct sunlight.

Standardization:

Test for bioactive compounds like withanolides to ensure therapeutic quality.

Quality Certifications:

Obtain certifications like USDA Organic or ISO to build consumer confidence.

Storage And Handling

"Preservation protects potential."

Proper storage ensures the longevity of Ashwagandha products, retaining potency and efficacy.

Tips for Storage:
Environment:

Store in a cool, dry place away from moisture and sunlight.

Packaging:

Use airtight, UV-resistant containers.

Labeling:

Clearly label with batch number and expiration date for traceability.

Ensuring Longevity of Products

"Sustainability lies in foresight."

Extend the shelf life of Ashwagandha products through these measures:

Use of Desiccants:
Place silica gel packets in packaging to absorb moisture.

Refrigeration:

For powdered products, refrigeration minimizes degradation.

Map And Diagram For Better Understanding

Below is an illustrative representation of the Ashwagandha growth and maintenance process:

Diagram: Ashwagandha Cultivation and Care

Planting

Shows seed placement and spacing.

Growth Stages

Seedlings to mature plants.

Harvesting and Drying

Highlight the root extraction process and drying techniques.

Stage	Activity	Requirements	Outcome
Planting	Seed sowing	Well-drained soil, 1 cm depth	Healthy seedlings

Watering	Weekly irrigation	Moderate water supply	Root development
Fertilizing	Compost addition	Organic nutrients	Enhanced growth
Pest Control	Neem oil spray	Eco-friendly pesticides	Disease-free plants

A Brief History Of Ashwagandha

Ashwagandha, translated as "smell of the horse," has been a cornerstone of Ayurvedic medicine for over 3,000 years. Its roots, symbolizing strength and vitality, were traditionally used to combat stress, improve sleep, and enhance immunity.

Relevant Websites:

National Center for Biotechnology Information (NCBI) – Detailed scientific studies on Ashwagandha.

Ayurveda.com – Insights on traditional Ayurvedic practices.

CHAPTER 6

The Ultimate Guide To Using Ashwagandha

Simple Steps For Beginners

Background and Brief History

Ashwagandha, also known as Withania somnifera or Indian Ginseng, has been a staple of Ayurvedic medicine for centuries. Known for its adaptogenic properties, it helps the body adapt to stress and promote overall balance.

Its origins trace back thousands of years in India, where it was considered a tonic for longevity, vitality, and rejuvenation. The name "Ashwagandha" comes from the Sanskrit words "ashva" (horse) and "gandha" (smell), referring to its potent odor and its ability to impart strength and vitality.

"Ashwagandha: a time-tested herb connecting ancient wisdom with modern health solutions."

Websites like AyurvedicHealing.com and HerbalGuide.org provide additional resources and scientific studies on Ashwagandha for deeper understanding.

Purpose Of Studying Ashwagandha

Studying Ashwagandha helps beginners unlock the herb's full potential, transitioning from casual use to becoming well-informed experts. Understanding its effects on stress, immunity, hormonal balance, and cognitive function ensures users can tailor its use for optimal health outcomes.

Identifying Your Goals

Before using Ashwagandha, identify your specific health objectives.

Stress Reduction: Use Ashwagandha for its calming properties.

Boosting Energy: Harness its ability to enhance vitality and stamina.

Enhancing Cognitive Function: Support focus and mental clarity.

"Every goal has a starting point. Let Ashwagandha become the cornerstone of your wellness journey."

Key Recipe Example:
Ashwagandha Stress Relief Tea

Ingredients: 1 tsp Ashwagandha powder, 1 cup warm water, 1 tsp honey, a pinch of cinnamon.

Preparation: Mix powder in warm water, add honey and cinnamon, and stir well.

Selecting the Right Product

Ashwagandha is available in various forms such as powders, capsules, tinctures, and teas. Look for:

Certified Organic: Free from harmful pesticides.

Third-Party Testing: Ensures potency and purity.

Type of Extraction: Choose KSM-66 or Sensoril for standardized potency.

Table Example:

Form	Benefits	Best Use
Powder	Versatile, can mix in drinks	Ideal for teas and smoothies
Capsules	Convenient, pre-measured dose	On-the-go supplementation
Tinctures	Fast-absorbing, potent	Quick relief for stress

Creating A Routine

To maximize benefits, integrate Ashwagandha into your daily routine. Use it consistently at the same time every day.

Morning Routine Example:
Wake Up Energy Drink

Blend 1 tsp Ashwagandha powder, 1 banana, 1 cup almond milk, and a dash of turmeric for a revitalizing smoothie.

Night Routine Example:
Calming Milk Elixir

Combine 1 cup warm milk (or plant-based alternative), 1 tsp Ashwagandha, and 1 tsp honey to unwind before bed.

Incorporating Ashwagandha into Lifestyle

Make Ashwagandha a part of your holistic wellness routine. Pair it with yoga, meditation, or a healthy diet for amplified effects.

"Balance is not something you find; it is something you create with intention."

Example Lifestyle Map:
Morning: Ashwagandha smoothie + light yoga.

Afternoon: Ashwagandha capsule + balanced lunch.

Evening: Calming Ashwagandha tea + meditation.

Recipes for Health, Skin, and Wellness

Ashwagandha can transform your skincare and wellness rituals. Rich in antioxidants, it promotes healthy, glowing skin and fights inflammation.

DIY Face Mask:
Ingredients: 1 tsp Ashwagandha powder, 1 tbsp yogurt, 1 tsp honey.

Instructions: Mix ingredients and apply to your face for 10–15 minutes. Rinse with warm water for a natural glow.

Wellness Tonic:
Mix 1 tsp Ashwagandha powder with warm water, lemon juice, and ginger for a detoxifying drink.

Morning Rituals With Ashwagandha

Start your day with grounding practices that include Ashwagandha for sustained energy and focus.

Recipe: Energizing Coffee Alternative

Ingredients: 1 cup chai tea, 1 tsp Ashwagandha powder, 1/2 tsp cardamom, 1 tsp honey.

Preparation: Mix the ingredients and enjoy warm.

Creative Ways to Use Ashwagandha

Move beyond teas and capsules by infusing Ashwagandha into unique recipes.

Ashwagandha Bliss Balls:
Ingredients: 1 cup dates, 1 cup almonds, 2 tbsp Ashwagandha powder, 1 tbsp cacao powder.

Preparation: Blend all ingredients into a paste, form small balls, and refrigerate.

Ashwagandha Pancakes:
Add 1 tsp Ashwagandha powder to your pancake mix for a nutritious breakfast boost.

Teas, Smoothies, and Powders

The versatility of Ashwagandha makes it ideal for beverages.

Soothing Night Tea:
Ingredients: Chamomile tea bag, 1 tsp Ashwagandha powder, and honey.

Preparation: Brew tea, stir in Ashwagandha, and sweeten with honey.

Ashwagandha can be a foundation for DIY health and beauty products.

Stress-Relief Bath Soak:
Mix 1 cup Epsom salt, 1 tbsp Ashwagandha powder, and 10 drops lavender essential oil for a calming soak.

Visual Aids for Understanding
Infographic: Integrating Ashwagandha into Daily Life

Morning: Smoothies and teas.

Afternoon: Capsules or tonics.

Evening: Relaxing milk elixirs and skincare rituals.

Diagram of the Ashwagandha Reproduction & Distribution Process:

Cultivation:
Grown in sandy soils with proper irrigation.

Root harvested after 5-6 months.

Processing:
Roots cleaned, dried, and ground into powder.

Distribution:
Packaged into capsules, tinctures, or powders for sale globally.

Stage	Action
Cultivation	Planting, irrigation, and care.
Harvesting	Collecting roots after maturity.

| Processing | Cleaning and grinding. |
| Packaging | Sealing for freshness. |

This detailed breakdown ensures beginners can understand and apply Ashwagandha effectively in their lives.

CHAPTER 7

Comparative Analysis

Understanding Artificial And Natural Ashwagandha

Ashwagandha, often referred to as "Indian Ginseng," is a revered herb in Ayurvedic medicine. But as modern practices evolve, so does its production. The market today offers two main forms: natural and artificial Ashwagandha.

Natural Ashwagandha is cultivated organically without synthetic chemicals. It's harvested from the roots and leaves of the Withania somnifera plant, ensuring its traditional potency and purity.

Artificial Ashwagandha, often manufactured in labs, uses synthetic compounds to mimic the herb's active constituents. While affordable and mass-produced, it lacks the holistic balance found in nature.

Recipes For Understanding

Infographic Example: A side-by-side comparison chart showing cultivation, production methods, benefits, and potential downsides of natural and artificial Ashwagandha.

Sample Image Concept: A field of sunlit Ashwagandha plants vs. a sterile laboratory setting with vials labeled "Ashwagandha Extract."

Nutritional Value And Potency

Unpacking Nutritional Profiles

Natural Ashwagandha contains a wealth of bioactive compounds:

Withanolides: Known for anti-inflammatory and anti-cancer properties.

Alkaloids: Stress-relieving and mood-enhancing agents.

Iron and Antioxidants: Essential for immunity and vitality.

Artificial Ashwagandha often isolates specific compounds, which can result in higher potency per dose but lacks the synergistic effects of natural extracts.

Recipes For Beginners

Natural Ashwagandha Tea:
Ingredients: 1 tsp Ashwagandha powder, 1 cup water, honey (optional).

Steps: Boil water, add powder, simmer for 5 minutes, strain, and sweeten if desired.

Artificial Ashwagandha Smoothie:
Ingredients: ½ tsp artificial Ashwagandha extract, banana, almond milk, and a handful of spinach.

Blend all ingredients until smooth. Ideal for quick energy.

Ethical Considerations

Challenges in Ethical Sourcing

Sourcing natural Ashwagandha raises concerns about:

Fair Trade Practices: Are farmers paid fairly?

Sustainability: Are crops grown without depleting local ecosystems?

Artificial Ashwagandha may sidestep these issues but introduces questions about environmental impact during chemical synthesis.

Practical Takeaways

Look for certifications like USDA Organic or Fair Trade.

Support local communities by purchasing from ethical brands.

Lessons from Artificial and Natural Products

What We Can Learn

Holistic Healing vs. Precision Dosing:

Natural Ashwagandha offers a broad spectrum of benefits but may take longer to work.

Artificial options cater to individuals needing rapid or targeted effects.

Cultural Connection:

Natural Ashwagandha ties us to ancient practices and traditions, a journey beyond mere consumption.

Examples:

Visual: A pie chart breaking down the benefits users seek (stress relief, sleep improvement, etc.).

Quote: "Nature teaches patience, while science teaches precision. Both have a place in the modern world."

Moral Implications In Sourcing

Deep Dive into the Moral Landscape
Harvesting Ashwagandha is not just a transaction; it's a relationship with nature:

Deforestation concerns from overharvesting.

Exploitation of farmers in developing regions.

The rise of eco-friendly lab production offers an alternative but must align with broader sustainability goals.

Practical Takeaways

Guiding Principles
Opt for transparency in labeling.

Prioritize sustainable packaging.

Educate yourself on brand commitments to ethics.

Actionable Recipe:
Ashwagandha Oil for Relaxation:

Ingredients: Organic Ashwagandha root, sesame oil, coconut oil.

Process: Heat oils gently, infuse with dried root for 3-4 hours, strain, and store in a glass bottle.

Generated Visual: Holistic Understanding

Diagram: Lifecycle of Ashwagandha Products

Natural Ashwagandha:

Cultivation → Traditional Harvesting → Minimal Processing → Consumer.

Artificial Ashwagandha:

Lab Cultivation → Chemical Extraction → Synthetic Production → Consumer.

Map Visual Example:

A flowchart connecting farming regions (India, Nepal) to global supply chains, emphasizing transparency.

Column Table Example: Comparing Artificial vs. Natural Ashwagandha

Aspect	Natural Ashwagandha	Artificial Ashwagandha
Production Method	Organic cultivation, hand-harvested	Lab-synthesized, industrial processes
Potency	Balanced bioactive compounds	Isolated, concentrated compounds
Sustainability	Risk of overharvesting, eco-friendly farming	Low agricultural impact but high energy use
Ethics	Dependent on fair trade practices	Controlled, less tied to traditional systems
Cost	Moderate to high	Often lower

Ashwagandha's roots trace back over 3,000 years in Ayurveda. Known for its adaptogenic properties, it was first documented in ancient Indian texts like the Charaka Samhita. Its name translates to "smell of a horse," symbolizing vitality and strength.

Website Example

A curated site like www.AshwagandhaWorld.com could include:

Educational blogs.

Ethical sourcing guides.

Recipe tutorials.

A shopping portal for certified natural and artificial Ashwagandha products.

Quote for Inspiration: "Every herb carries a story of the earth; in Ashwagandha, we find strength rooted in tradition and shaped by science."

CHAPTER 8

Rules For Success In The Ashwagandha Craft Business

Brief History Of Ashwagandha

Ashwagandha (Withania somnifera), a cornerstone of Ayurvedic medicine, has been revered for over 3,000 years.

It is known as the "Indian Ginseng" for its rejuvenating properties and translates to "smell of the horse," indicating its potential to impart the vigor and strength of a stallion. Originating in India, this adaptogenic herb has gained global recognition for its ability to combat stress, improve focus, and boost overall well-being.

Today, Ashwagandha is cultivated primarily in India but is also distributed in Africa, the Middle East, and parts of Asia.

The herb is made available in various forms, including powders, capsules, teas, and tinctures, making it accessible for both health practitioners and consumers worldwide.

Website Suggestion for History and Insights:
For additional information, visit AshwagandhaCraft.com, a resource hub for the cultivation, benefits, and applications of Ashwagandha.

Rules For Success In The Ashwagandha Craft Business

Rules for Starting and Succeeding

Understand the Market: Conduct in-depth research to understand demand trends, target demographics, and global popularity of Ashwagandha products.

Identify Your Niche: Determine if you will focus on health supplements, beverages, skincare, or other innovative uses for Ashwagandha.

Develop High-Quality Products: Emphasize organic and sustainable farming practices to ensure premium-quality offerings.

Leverage Storytelling: Share the cultural and historical relevance of Ashwagandha to connect with your audience on a personal level.

Importance of Research

Deep research is the foundation of success in the Ashwagandha business. It ensures:

Understanding customer needs and expectations.

Analyzing competitors' strategies and differentiating yourself.

Identifying potential markets for expansion.

Example Research Plan:

Step	Action	Tool

1	Study market trends	Google Trends, MarketWatch
2	Analyze competitors	SWOT Analysis
3	Survey target audiences	Online Surveys

Building A Unique Selling Proposition (USP)

Your USP is what makes your Ashwagandha products stand out. Focus on:

Health Benefits: Emphasize purity, effectiveness, and health impact.

Sustainability: Highlight eco-friendly production practices.

Authenticity: Connect your product to its Ayurvedic roots.

Example Recipe for USP:

Ingredient	Action
Organic sourcing	Partner with certified farmers
Scientific validation	Invest in clinical studies
Storytelling	Craft narratives around benefits

Creating Strong Customer Relationships

Developing lasting relationships requires:
Transparent communication about product ingredients and benefits.

Educating customers on the proper use of Ashwagandha through blogs, webinars, or eBooks.

Building loyalty programs for repeat customers.

Recipe for Strong Relationships:

Ingredient	Example
Trust	Share test reports and customer testimonials
Accessibility	Ensure easy ordering and excellent support
Engagement	Regular newsletters with health tips

Maintaining Ethical Standards

Ethics build trust and credibility. To achieve this:

Source sustainably to protect the environment.

Ensure fair wages for farmers and workers.

Avoid misleading claims about product capabilities.

How To Ponder Over Challenges In Business

Strategies for Problem-Solving

SWOT Analysis: Regularly review strengths, weaknesses, opportunities, and threats.

Collaborations: Partner with like-minded businesses to expand reach.

Risk Management: Invest in insurance and diversification.

Ensuring Flexibility

Stay agile to adapt to market shifts, including the demand for new product formats like gummies, infused oils, or Ashwagandha-enriched snacks.

Visual Guide: Ashwagandha Business Success Map

Key Components of Success Map:
Cultivation & Sourcing: Use organic soil and non-GMO seeds.

Production Process: Adhere to GMP standards for safety and efficacy.

Distribution Channels: Partner with e-commerce platforms, wellness stores, and local markets.

Marketing Strategies: Utilize SEO, social media, and influencer collaborations.

Column Table for Summary

Aspect	Key Points	Example
Research	Understand demand and competitors	Survey customers about preferences
USP	Highlight benefits and authenticity	Market as "organic" and "traditionally crafted"
Ethical Standards	Sustainable farming, fair wages	Use eco-friendly packaging
Customer Relationships	Engage and educate	Offer a free eBook on Ashwagandha benefits
Flexibility	Adapt to market trends	Introduce gummies alongside powders

"Success in the Ashwagandha craft business lies in a blend of tradition, innovation, and integrity. Build with care, and the world will trust your roots."

CHAPTER 9

The Economic Impact Of Ashwagandha

Ashwagandha (Withania somnifera), commonly known as "Indian ginseng," has a rich history deeply rooted in Ayurvedic medicine and has recently gained global attention due to its numerous health benefits.

However, its significance extends far beyond its medicinal properties; Ashwagandha plays a pivotal role in economic development, food security, and sustainability.

As the world turns toward more sustainable and natural health solutions, Ashwagandha has emerged as a vital crop with the potential to shape economies and improve livelihoods. This section will delve into how Ashwagandha impacts the economy, its role in food security, financial prospects, and the sustainability of agricultural practices.

Ashwagandha As An Economic Crop

Historical Context of Ashwagandha Cultivation
Ashwagandha has been cultivated for thousands of years in India, where it was primarily used in traditional Ayurvedic medicine.

Historically, it was grown in arid and semi-arid regions of India, where its adaptability to harsh conditions made it a valuable crop. Over time, Ashwagandha cultivation spread to other parts of the world, with the crop now growing in many countries, including the Middle East, parts of Africa, and North America.

The demand for Ashwagandha in the global market is on the rise, with its roots, leaves, and seeds being used in supplements, beverages, skincare products, and more.

Economic Contribution

The cultivation of Ashwagandha provides economic benefits at various levels, from small-scale farmers to large-scale industrial producers. As a hardy crop, it requires minimal water and grows in poor soil, making it an attractive option for farmers, especially in regions facing water scarcity.

The global market for Ashwagandha is estimated to grow at a significant rate, driven by increased demand for natural health products. This growing market creates income opportunities for farmers, processors, and exporters.

Role In Food Security

Ashwagandha as a Nutritional Supplement

While primarily known for its medicinal properties, Ashwagandha also has nutritional benefits that can contribute to food security.

Ashwagandha roots are rich in bioactive compounds that have been shown to support overall health, reduce stress, and enhance immunity. In regions where malnutrition is prevalent, Ashwagandha could be integrated into dietary supplements or functional foods, improving the health and well-being of vulnerable populations.

Cultivation and Resilience

Due to its resilience in challenging environments, Ashwagandha is an important crop for maintaining food security in areas affected by drought or erratic weather patterns. Its ability to thrive in low-resource environments makes it a reliable crop for smallholder farmers, ensuring stable production even under adverse conditions.

Financial Prospects

Economic Growth And Job Creation

The increasing demand for Ashwagandha-based products opens up significant financial prospects, particularly for developing countries. From cultivation to manufacturing to retail, Ashwagandha supports a variety of industries and creates job opportunities across the supply chain.

As the global demand for herbal supplements, functional foods, and organic products rises, Ashwagandha offers a lucrative market for farmers, entrepreneurs, and businesses alike.

Export Opportunities

Ashwagandha is one of the most sought-after herbs in the global market, especially in the United States, Europe, and other Western countries. Exporting Ashwagandha products can be a profitable venture for countries like India, where the crop is grown extensively.

By tapping into this international demand, countries can enhance their economic standing while promoting local agriculture and sustainable practices.

Ashwagandha and Sustainability

Environmental Benefits Of Ashwagandha Cultivation

Ashwagandha is considered a sustainable crop due to its low water requirements and ability to grow in poor soil conditions.

Unlike many cash crops that deplete the soil and require significant irrigation, Ashwagandha is a hardy plant that can be grown with minimal environmental impact. This makes it an ideal choice for sustainable farming practices, especially in regions affected by climate change and resource scarcity.

Supporting Biodiversity And Soil Health

Cultivating Ashwagandha also promotes biodiversity. Its cultivation does not rely heavily on synthetic fertilizers or pesticides, thus reducing the impact on the surrounding ecosystem. Moreover, because Ashwagandha is often grown as a rotational crop, it can contribute to the restoration of soil health, improving the long-term sustainability of farming systems.

Supporting Local Economies

Empowering Small-Scale Farmers

For small-scale farmers, Ashwagandha provides a means to diversify income sources. By growing a high-value crop that requires relatively little investment and maintenance, farmers can improve their financial stability and secure better livelihoods for their families.

The growing popularity of Ashwagandha also helps small-scale producers integrate into the global market, allowing them to sell their products at competitive prices.

Community Development
The expansion of Ashwagandha cultivation can positively impact rural communities by creating jobs in farming, processing, and distribution. Local economies can flourish as a result of increased demand, and rural areas can become hubs for Ashwagandha-related industries, further contributing to national economic growth.

Recipes and Usage
Ashwagandha can be consumed in various forms. Here are some simple ways to incorporate Ashwagandha into your daily life:

Ashwagandha Powder Milk
Ingredients:

1 cup of warm milk

1 tsp of Ashwagandha powder

Honey or sweetener (optional)

Directions:

Mix the Ashwagandha powder into warm milk and stir well.

Add honey or sweetener if desired.

Drink before bed to promote restful sleep and reduce stress.

Ashwagandha Smoothie
Ingredients:

1 banana

1/2 cup of yogurt or almond milk

1 tsp of Ashwagandha powder

1 tsp of honey

Directions:
Blend all ingredients until smooth.

Drink in the morning to boost energy levels and enhance mental clarity.

Background And Purpose Of Studying Ashwagandha

The study of Ashwagandha provides valuable insights into its economic potential and health benefits. By understanding the history of Ashwagandha cultivation, its medicinal properties, and its role in modern agriculture, researchers can uncover innovative ways to integrate Ashwagandha into global markets while promoting sustainable farming practices.

Aspiring experts in this field can contribute to the advancement of this ancient crop, helping to harness its potential for both health and economic growth.

Purpose Of Studying Ashwagandha

Health Applications: Researchers aim to understand how Ashwagandha can help treat chronic stress, anxiety, and improve physical performance.

Agricultural Innovation: Scientists study how Ashwagandha can be cultivated more efficiently, sustainably, and in various climates.

Market Expansion: As the demand for herbal products grows, understanding the economic impact and potential for Ashwagandha cultivation is crucial.

Reproduction And Distribution Process

Ashwagandha cultivation involves several stages, from seed production to harvesting and distribution. The process includes the following steps:

Seed Selection: Choosing high-quality seeds from reliable sources.

Cultivation: Preparing the soil and planting Ashwagandha in optimal conditions.

Harvesting: Timing the harvest when the roots are at their most potent.

Processing: Drying and grinding the roots into powder or extracts.

Distribution: Transporting Ashwagandha products to local and international markets.

"Ashwagandha is not just a crop; it is a bridge between ancient wisdom and modern sustainability. It provides not only health but also hope, for individuals, for communities, and for the world."

Visual Representation Of Ashwagandha's Economic Impact

Below is a conceptual diagram that illustrates the relationship between Ashwagandha cultivation, economic growth, and environmental sustainability.

Table: Economic Impact of Ashwagandha

Category	Impact	Details
Economic Crop	High-value cash crop	Contributes to local and national economies through farming and exports.
Role in Food Security	Nutritional benefits	Can be used in supplements, aiding in improving health in food-insecure areas.
Financial Prospects	Job creation and income generation	Opportunities in farming, processing, and export.

Sustainability	Low environmental impact	Requires minimal water and is grown in poor soil conditions.
Supporting Local Economies	Empowering small-scale farmers	Provides income and promotes economic stability in rural areas.

By incorporating these elements into your understanding, this guide helps readers see the full potential of Ashwagandha, not only as a powerful herb for health but also as a key player in the global economic landscape.

CHAPTER 10

Health And Wellness Through Ashwagandha

Ashwagandha, often referred to as "Indian ginseng" or "winter cherry," has been revered for centuries in traditional Ayurvedic medicine. Its profound impact on overall health, mental clarity, and physical vitality makes it a powerful ally for enhancing wellness.

This chapter delves deep into Ashwagandha's extraordinary potential to nurture both body and mind, offering scientifically-backed insights and practical applications for beginners.

Enhancing Innate And Adaptive Immunity

Ashwagandha has long been known for its remarkable ability to support immune function. Through its adaptogenic properties, it helps the body adapt to stress while boosting both innate and adaptive immunity.

Innate Immunity: Ashwagandha enhances the first line of defense by supporting the body's natural barriers, such as the skin and mucous membranes, and promoting the activity of immune cells like macrophages and neutrophils.

Adaptive Immunity: It also aids the second line of defense by improving the body's ability to recognize and remember specific pathogens. Ashwagandha modulates the function of T-cells, B-cells, and natural killer (NK) cells, helping the immune system recognize threats more effectively.

Scientific Insights And Research

Recent studies highlight Ashwagandha's potent immune-modulating effects. For example, a study published in Phytotherapy Research showed that Ashwagandha supplementation significantly improved the levels of antioxidants in the body, thereby promoting better immune function.

Furthermore, the root of Ashwagandha contains withanolides, compounds shown to modulate inflammation and oxidative stress, key factors that influence immune health.

Practical Applications

Ashwagandha can be incorporated into daily life in several ways. To boost immunity, it can be consumed in various forms such as:

Ashwagandha powder: Mix with warm water or add it to smoothies.

Ashwagandha capsules or tablets: These are a convenient option for those who prefer a precise dosage.

Ashwagandha tea: Brewed with ginger and honey for a soothing, immune-boosting drink.

Recipes for Wellness

Ashwagandha Water:

A simple yet effective drink for boosting immunity and calming the mind.

Ingredients:
1 tsp Ashwagandha powder

1 cup warm water

Honey or lemon (optional)

Instructions:
Mix Ashwagandha powder in warm water. Stir well.

Drink once a day in the morning or before bed for maximum benefits.

Smoothies and Blends:
For a more refreshing and nutritious way to incorporate Ashwagandha, try these smoothie recipes.

Ashwagandha Mango Smoothie:
Ingredients:

1 cup mango

1 tsp Ashwagandha powder

1 tbsp honey

1 cup almond milk or coconut water

A pinch of turmeric

Instructions:
Blend all ingredients until smooth. Drink in the morning for an energy boost.

Ashwagandha Chocolate Almond Smoothie:
Ingredients:

1 cup almond milk

1 tbsp almond butter

1 tsp Ashwagandha powder

1 tbsp cocoa powder

1 banana

Ice cubes

Instructions:
Blend all ingredients until creamy and smooth. Enjoy as a post-workout recovery smoothie.

Purpose Of Studying To Become An Expert

Understanding Ashwagandha's full potential requires knowledge of its history, chemical composition, and how it interacts with various bodily systems. Studying Ashwagandha allows one to become an expert in leveraging this adaptogen for health benefits.

As with any natural remedy, it's essential to know the right dosage, potential side effects, and how it can complement other treatments. A comprehensive understanding will help you safely incorporate it into your lifestyle for optimal wellness.

Reproduction & Distribution Process

Ashwagandha's cultivation and distribution have been primarily within regions of India, Sri Lanka, and parts of Africa. The plant thrives in dry, arid climates, where it grows best in well-drained soil.

The roots of the plant are harvested and dried, then processed into powder or extract forms for distribution. The growing interest in herbal supplements has led to a widespread availability of Ashwagandha in various forms, from powders to capsules, across health food stores and online platforms.

The distribution process ensures that Ashwagandha reaches global markets, but it is crucial to source products from reputable suppliers to ensure the purity and potency of the plant. Authenticity is vital in maintaining the effectiveness of Ashwagandha supplements.

Example Of Ashwagandha Use:

Case Study:

Maria, a 32-year-old woman, had been feeling overwhelmed due to work stress. After consulting with her healthcare provider, she began incorporating Ashwagandha into her daily routine. She started with a simple Ashwagandha water recipe every morning. Within a few weeks, she noticed a reduction in her anxiety levels and improved focus at work.

Her immune system also seemed to be stronger, as she was less prone to catching colds.

By combining Ashwagandha with a balanced diet and regular exercise, Maria experienced a significant improvement in her overall well-being.

Column Table of Key Benefits and Uses of Ashwagandha

Benefit	Scientific Insight	Practical Application	Recipe Ideas
Stress Reductio n	Ashwagandh a reduces cortisol levels, helping the body cope with stress.	Add Ashwagandh a powder to warm water or smoothies.	Ashwagandh a Tea or Smoothie
Boosting Immunity	It enhances immune function through its antioxidant and anti-inflammatory properties.	Consume Ashwagandh a in powder form with honey for immune support.	Ashwagandh a Water or Mango Smoothie
Enhanced Focus & Clarity	Ashwagandh a is known to improve cognitive function and mental clarity.	Take Ashwagandh a capsules or use powder in your daily drinks.	Ashwagandh a Chocolate Almond Smoothie

Physical Vitality	It promotes energy and reduces fatigue by balancing energy levels.	Incorporate into morning smoothies for an energy boost.	Mango and Ashwagandha Smoothie

Diagram Or Map

Below is a simplified conceptual map showing how Ashwagandha works to support different areas of health.

Ashwagandha's Impact on Stress and Immunity:
Stress Reduction → Lower Cortisol Levels → Better Immune Function

Adaptogen Action → Enhanced Physical Vitality

Antioxidants → Reduced Inflammation → Strengthened Body Defenses

Ashwagandha's Role in Mental Clarity and Focus:
Cognitive Boost → Enhanced Focus

Anti-fatigue → Improved Physical Energy

Mood Stabilizer → Reduced Anxiety

By understanding these elements—scientific insights, practical applications, and the variety of recipes that incorporate Ashwagandha—you are well on your way to mastering the art of using this herb to improve your health and wellness.

As you become familiar with its uses and effects, Ashwagandha will become an indispensable part of your health regimen.

CONCLUSION

The conclusion of the matter encapsulates the holistic journey through the world of Ashwagandha, revealing its profound significance for beginners, enthusiasts, and entrepreneurs alike.

Rooted in centuries of cultural reverence and modern-day scientific validation, Ashwagandha emerges as a versatile and impactful herb with a spectrum of benefits. From stress relief, improved sleep, and hormonal balance to supporting mental, physical, and cognitive health, it holds a pivotal place in wellness routines.

Beginners are advised to navigate challenges mindfully, avoiding misuse and adhering to safety practices, while business aspirants are encouraged to explore sustainable opportunities through creative ventures like Ashwagandha craft businesses.

Through chapters detailing its natural and artificial forms, botanical intricacies, cultivation, and product development, the narrative bridges traditional knowledge and contemporary applications. Moreover, insights into the ethical, nutritional, and economic aspects underscore Ashwagandha's global relevance.

Its adaptability shines in diverse formats—teas, smoothies, skincare products—making it a staple for holistic living.

Whether embraced as a personal remedy or a business foundation, the journey with Ashwagandha promises wellness, sustainability, and innovation, marking it as not just a herb but a transformative asset in health and commerce.